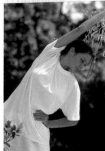

healing
energies

Using the powers

of nature to heal

mind, body and spirit

Raje Airey

HERMES
HOUSE

The edition published by Hermes House

© Anness Publishing Limited 2002 updated 2003..

Hermes House is an imprint of Anness Publishing Limited,
Hermes House, 88–89 Blackfriars Road, London SE1 8HA

Publisher: Joanna Lorenz
Production Controller: Joanna King

Publisher's Note:
The Reader should not regard the recommendations, ideas and techniques
expressed and described in this book as substitutes for the advice of a
qualified medical practitioner or other qualified professional.
Any use to which the recommendations, ideas and techniques
are put is at the reader's sole discretion and risk.

Printed in Hong Kong/China

3 5 7 9 10 8 6 4

contents

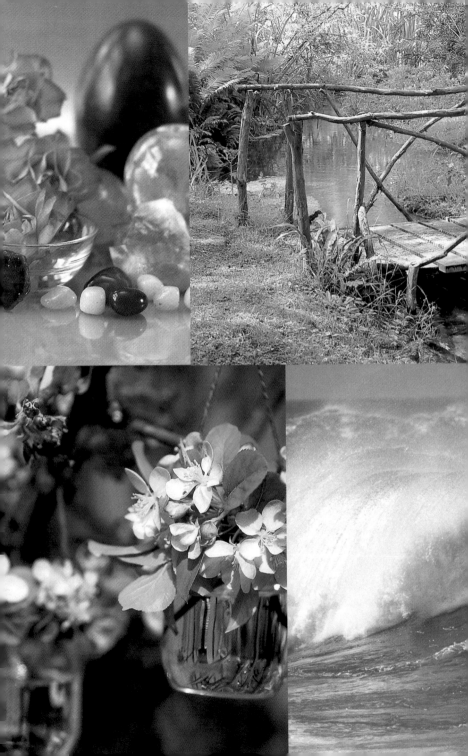

introduction

Healing with energy is as old as humankind. The techniques that tap into invisible energy forces include working with subtle vibrations of colour, light and sound, harnessing the energies of plants and minerals, and understanding the cosmic energies of the sun and moon. This book explains how to diagnose and treat energy imbalances using both ancient and modern methods, from acupuncture and feng shui to Vega testing and radionics. It also describes how energy therapies can help with common health problems, including chronic fatigue, allergies and emotional stress, and for pain relief.

what is energy?

Energy is life. It is the invisible force that animates the human body and permeates everything in the natural world, including animals, plants, trees and rocks, as well as the earth, sun, moon and stars.

THE LIFE FORCE

Throughout the course of history, cultures all over the world have acknowledged the existence of a universal energy force flowing through everything in the world, including the human body. It has been given many names. In India it is referred to as "prana", in the Far East it is "chi" or "ki", while in some shamanist traditions it is described as "chula" or "animu". Today, many people refer to it as "spirit" or the "life force".

Invisible like the air we breathe, the life force has a powerful influence on our health and wellbeing. It not only governs our physical health and survival, but it is also responsible for our mental and emotional wellbeing; it is the spark that fuels our ambitions, driving us to express our personal creativity and strive to fulfil our spiritual potential.

Good health is achieved when the life force is balanced and allowed to flow freely. When it is blocked or unbalanced, it leads to disturbances that will eventually manifest as "dis-ease" or a state of disharmony in the natural order. Energy healing is all about finding ways to strengthen, balance and free up this energy by using naturally occurring vibrations, such as light or colour, or the energies of natural forms such as plants and crystals.

▼ A MASSIVE TREE STARTS LIFE AS A SEED THAT IS PULSING WITH LIFE FORCE ENERGY AS WELL AS THE POTENTIAL FOR GROWTH.

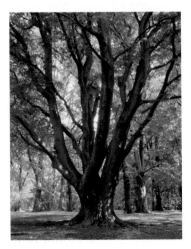

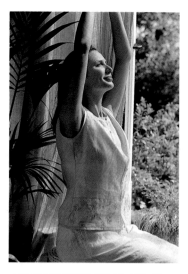

▲ WHEN THE LIFE FORCE IS IN HARMONY YOU FEEL READY TO TAKE ON THE WORLD.

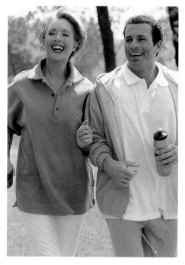

▲ BY TAPPING INTO NATURE'S HEALING ENERGY WE CAN BE FILLED WITH WELLBEING.

A UNIVERSE OF ENERGY

The life force connects us to the world we live in, weaving the fabric of life seamlessly together. Everything within the universe vibrates with energy and the world that we are part of is a vast web of energy patterns.

This idea has been verified by modern science. All matter, however dense it may appear, is made up of energy: it consists of atoms, protons, neutrons, electrons, waves and particles, all vibrating together at different frequencies. We live in the electromagnetic energy field of the earth, surrounded by wave forms, from low frequency radio waves at one end of the spectrum to high frequency cosmic rays at the other. Everything in the universe is made up of energy, which becomes more dense (and vibrates at a lower frequency) as it forms into matter. We are energetic phenomena and our world is dynamic. Like everything else in our lives, our health is influenced by the invisible energies that flow through us and swirl all around us.

cosmic influences

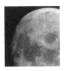

We are part of the cosmic web of life delicately connected and held in balance by subtle energy forces. Changes in any part of this energy system will have a "knock-on" effect on our health and vitality – for better or worse.

THE SUN

At the centre of our solar system, the sun is a fireball of light and heat, and is our most important energy source. It creates the conditions for life on earth and influences our health and vitality. When someone is sick, it is as though their "light" has dimmed. The word "influenza" comes from an Italian word meaning "to influence", and research indicates that all the major flu epidemics of the last 250 years (including the 1918 flu pandemic) have coincided with increased solar activity.

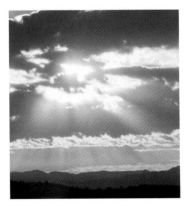

THE MOON

Lunar power controls the tides, affects weather, and influences human moods and behaviour. A woman's 28-day menstrual cycle follows the phases of the moon. The moon is also associated with psychological disturbances: the full moon is known as the time of lunacy or "moon madness", and its powerful energy can trigger such problems as epileptic fits, as well as increasing the potential for accidents.

BIORHYTHMS

The forces of the sun and the moon are often thought of as masculine and feminine energies respectively. The male solar energy is focused on action in the world outside, on ambition and achievement, while the female lunar energy is inwardly focused,

◀ BECAUSE THE SUN IS SO CRITICAL TO LIFE, IT WAS HELD IN AWE BY MANY EARLY CIVILIZATIONS AND REVERED AS A GOD. EVEN TODAY, PEOPLE DESCRIBE THEMSELVES AS "SUN-WORSHIPPERS".

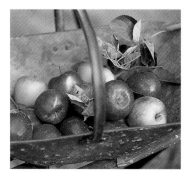

◄ COLLECTING APPLES AT HARVEST TIME REMINDS US OF NATURE'S CYCLES AND THE CHANGING SEASONS OF THE YEAR.

world", while at other times we feel lethargic and find it more difficult to get things done.

THE SEASONS

The changing seasons also affect our energy levels and many illnesses are seasonal. Light deprivation is thought to be associated with seasonal affective disorder (SAD), which is a severe manifestation of the "winter blues". We suffer more colds and flu in winter, whereas early summer is the hayfever season.

and more concerned with the intuitive world of feelings and emotion. According to the theory of biorhythms, we all have an internal male "solar" cycle and a female "lunar" cycle that affects us physically, emotionally and intellectually. These cycles produce a pattern of highs and lows, so that some days we may have lots of energy and feel "on top of the

▼ BOTH MEN AND WOMEN CONTAIN A BALANCE OF FEMININE AND MASCULINE ENERGIES, ALSO KNOWN AS YIN AND YANG.

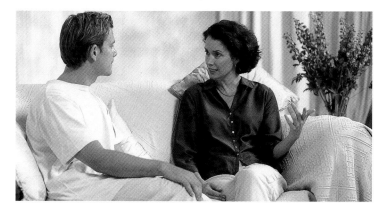

the human energy field

There is more to the human form than meets the eye. The vital force emanates around the body like a luminous sphere or "aura", entering through the chakras and running along energy pathways, or meridians.

THE AURA

The body's aura is subtle energy that vibrates at a different wavelength and frequency to the energy of the physical body. It is sometimes seen or depicted as a halo and may be felt when someone "enters your space". Auras vary in size, density and colour, but their overall size, shape and vibrancy is indicative of your state of health. The healthier you are, the larger and brighter your aura; when you are sick, your aura contracts as the body tries to conserve its vital energy. The size of the aura can also depend on mood and place.

SUBTLE ANATOMY

The energy pod around the human form can be visualized as seven layers of light, each vibrating at a higher frequency than the previous one. These layers are also known as the

THE SUBTLE BODIES

1 Etheric body: closest to the physical body; provides a blueprint for the physical body and its organs.
2 Emotional body: the seat of the emotions.
3 Mental body: mental activity, thoughts, ideas and day-to-day concerns.
4 Astral body: represents the personality.
5 Causal body: seat of willpower and gateway to higher consciousness; fulfilment of personal destiny.
6 Celestial soul body: spiritual essence, sometimes referred to as the "higher self".
7 Illuminated spiritual body: the highest and most refined level, where we become one with the source of love and healing, or the Divine.

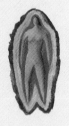

▲ WE ARE AWARE OF HUMAN ENERGY FIELDS WHEN WE SENSE THE MOOD OF SOMEONE CLOSE BY, OR FEEL OUR "SPACE" IS INVADED WHEN SOMEONE COMES TOO NEAR US.

7TH THE CROWN CHAKRA STIMULATES PERCEPTION AND INTUITION AND MAINTAINS THE OVERALL BALANCE OF THE SYSTEM.

6TH THE BROW CHAKRA (THIRD EYE) IS CONCERNED WITH UNDERSTANDING AND MENTAL ORGANIZATION.

5TH THE THROAT CHAKRA GOVERNS COMMUNICATION, EXPRESSION AND THE FLOW OF INFORMATION.

4TH THE HEART CHAKRA GOVERNS RELATIONSHIPS, PERSONAL DEVELOPMENT, JUDGMENT AND COMPASSION.

3RD THE SOLAR PLEXUS CHAKRA IS CONCERNED WITH SELF-CONFIDENCE AS WELL AS PERSONAL POWER.

2ND THE SACRAL CHAKRA GOVERNS CREATIVITY, SEXUAL DRIVE AND PASSION.

1ST THE ROOT CHAKRA IS LINKED WITH PHYSICAL SURVIVAL, ENERGY DISTRIBUTION AND PRACTICALITY.

THE SEVEN CHAKRAS OR ENERGY CENTRES OF THE BODY ARE DEPICTED AS WHIRLING WHEELS OF COLOUR.

"subtle bodies", and each one has a special function. The energy of the subtle bodies enters and leaves the body through the chakras. It moves through the body along energy channels, called "nadis" or "meridians".

Health problems can arise when energy in the subtle bodies or chakras becomes congested or is under- or over-stimulated. The etheric body, for example, can become "muddied" by eating the wrong foods, and through lack of exercise. Or when it is not linked properly to the physical body, you are likely to experience low energy and persistent tiredness. Problems in one body or chakra can also have a knock-on effect on the others. Energy healing aims to bring the subtle bodies and the chakras into alignment. During any healing process, health and balance is understood to return to the subtle bodies first. Once the vibrational pattern is restored, the physical body then returns to health at its own slightly slower pace.

energy and health

Good health is achieved when our energy levels are in a state of balance. When they are depleted or out of balance, we become sick and unhappy. Living in balance and coping with change is the key to health.

ENERGY BALANCING

Chronic illnesses are on the increase, yet we tend to take our health for granted, paying attention only when something goes wrong. As we strive to meet the pressures of modern living, we push beyond our limits and "run on empty". We need to achieve a balance between the quality and quantity of the energy we give out and what we take in. This means balancing work and leisure, rest and exercise, and ensuring we have enough sleep and eat a balanced diet. If we take in too much of the "wrong" sort of energy, our systems become clogged up or blocked. This creates imbalance, first in the "subtle bodies" (layers of energy around the body), and eventually in the physical body.

THE EFFECTS OF STRESS

Many illnesses are stress-related, including digestive disorders such as irritable bowel syndrome (IBS), allergic conditions such as asthma, high blood pressure and "everyday" tension headaches. Stress is one of the biggest causes of energy imbalance; it affects us in many ways and at many levels. Negative mental and emotional states, such as anxiety, grief, fear, anger, worry and also depression, create turbulence in the subtle energy bodies and will lead to physical complaints if the imbalances are not corrected.

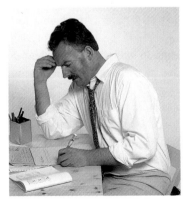

◀ OVERWORK CAN LEAD TO MENTAL AND EMOTIONAL STRESS, WHICH AFFECTS RELATIONSHIPS AND CAUSES HEALTH PROBLEMS.

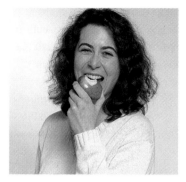

▲ WHEN YOU BITE INTO A FRESHLY PICKED ORGANIC APPLE, YOU CAN TELL THAT IT IS BURSTING WITH VITAL ENERGY.

▲ KEEP A PLANT ON YOUR DESK TO HELP PROTECT YOU FROM THE NEGATIVE ENERGIES CREATED BY ELECTRONIC OFFICE EQUIPMENT.

We are also affected by "geopathic stress", which is related to the electromagnetic energy fields of the earth. One natural cause of variations in the earth's energy field are underground water courses or "black streams". These have been thought to cause ill health for centuries. Indeed, recent research has associated them with chronic fatigue syndrome (ME), although the energy waves of modern electrical appliances, such as televisions, microwave ovens, computers and mobile phones, are also disturbing the earth's energy field, and may, in fact, be contributing to "modern" illnesses, such as ME, in ways that we don't yet understand.

COPING WITH CHANGE

Any point of change, or transition, is a critical time in life. This can be anything from a change in your personal lifestyle (such as getting divorced or married, changing job, having children, or moving house) to the changing seasons of the year or climate changes when we go abroad.

At a time of transition we should try to take extra care of ourselves, as the immune system is under increased pressure while we are attempting to adjust to a new or difficult situation. If we pay insufficient attention to our energy levels and carry on as though we are invincible, we will eventually get sick.

taking care of yourself

Your vital energy is your most precious commodity, and is worth looking after. For health and wellbeing, tune in to your energy field and learn to recognize the things that increase your energy levels and those that drain you.

ENERGY DRAINERS AND BOOSTERS
Take a good look at your lifestyle and use this guide to help you avoid the energy drainers and cultivate the energy boosters.

Key x = energy drainers
    ✓ = energy boosters
    ● = tip

FOOD AND DRINK
At the most basic level, food and drink is the fuel our bodies need in order to function. The closer it is to its natural, unrefined state, the greater the energy boost.

x Refined, processed food, white flour, sugar, alcohol, caffeine, "ready" meals, microwaved food.

✓ Raw food, unsweetened fresh fruit and vegetable juices, sprouted grains and seeds, freshly picked salad, fruit, vegetables.

● Drink 6 to 8 glasses of still mineral water a day. This will help to keep your system free of toxins.

RELATIONSHIPS
The people in our lives can be our greatest source of pleasure, yet they can also be a major cause of energy depletion. Some relationships are unavoidable, but with others you can be more selective.

x People who don't listen, have no time for you, "take" but don't give, tell you what to do/put you down/criticize you.

✓ People who make you laugh and feel good, share the balance of power, listen, are appreciative and supportive.

● Have a satisfying sex life.

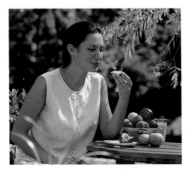

◀ MAKE SURE YOUR DIET INCLUDES PLENTY OF ENERGY-BOOSTING FOODS, SUCH AS FRESH FRUIT AND VEGETABLES.

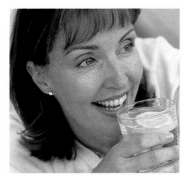

▲ AIM TO DRINK 6 TO 8 GLASSES OF WATER EVERY DAY TO CLEAR YOUR SYSTEM.

WORK

Since work is a major part of life, it's very important to find a way of working that suits you.

✗ Working long hours, not getting paid enough, "putting up with it", feeling forced to do it, lack of recognition.

✓ Enjoying what you do, getting a proper reward and recognition.

● Try to make your work fit around you and your needs; don't be a "wage slave".

> ### TIP
> Chronic illnesses are on the increase. Improve your resistance to disease by improving your energy levels. This will also help you to deal with any existing illness.

LIFESTYLE

Aim for balance in your activities and avoid going to extremes.

✗ Lack of sleep, exercise.

✓ Regular exercise and/or stress-reducing techniques, such as yoga, pilates, meditation, tai chi, working out.

● Make time for yourself each day.

ENVIRONMENT

Our surroundings have an instant effect on our energy levels.

✗ Packed city streets, busy shops, fluorescent lighting, clutter, lack of natural light and greenery.

✓ Nature, especially green leafy forests or windswept beaches, décor that makes you feel good, clear and tidy work spaces.

● Relax under a large leafy tree.

▼ TAKE REGULAR EXERCISE. GENTLE STRETCHING HELPS TO RELEASE TENSION.

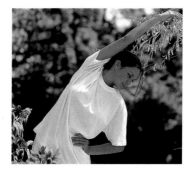

technology and energy

Technological advances in the 20th century have made it possible to measure the electrical energy fields of the human body. Kirlian photography and Vega testing both monitor energy patterns, using them for diagnosis.

KIRLIAN PHOTOGRAPHY

In 1939, Semyon Kirlian, a Russian electrician, discovered a way of producing an image of the electromagnetic energy field that surrounds the human body. To take a Kirlian photograph, the body's electromagnetic field (usually via the hands and/or feet) is brought into contact with a high-voltage, high-frequency electric charge. A photograph is taken of the resulting "interference pattern". This pattern can then be used to detect the strength or weakness of the body's electrical energy field, and shows where it is out of balance. A healthy body is indicated by a regular, bright field around the hand or foot, whereas a thin, patchy field indicates energy blocks or disturbances.

The pattern is affected by physical and emotional states. For instance, if you are in shock or exhausted, the energy pattern may not register, whereas if you are anxious or irritable, the image may have an erratic outer edge, with sharp points, rather than a smooth, even contour. The menstrual cycle, medication, as well as chronic or life-threatening illnesses such as cancer, also affect the energy pattern. Taking exercise, having acupuncture or other "energy-based medicines", meditating or doing yoga have all been shown to increase the radiance of the Kirlian image.

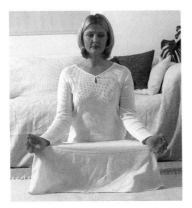

◄ KIRLIAN PHOTOGRAPHY IS ABLE TO DEMONSTRATE THAT THE AURA INCREASES IN SIZE AND RADIANCE DURING MEDITATION.

Vega testing

Research in Germany during the 1950s showed that acupuncture points on the body (where energy is concentrated and linked to specific organs) had electrical properties. Various electronic devices were then developed to measure and map these points, including the Vega machine, which was developed by Dr Helmut Schimmel in the 1970s.

Vega testing is used as a diagnostic technique, particularly to detect allergies or intolerances. During a Vega-testing consultation, an electronic probe or stylus is placed on certain points, usually on the feet and/or hands, while you hold an electrode in order to complete the circuit. The machine

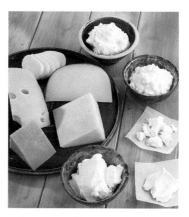

▲ ALLERGIES, OR OVER-SENSITIVITY TO CERTAIN FOODS, SUCH AS DAIRY PRODUCTS, ARE BECOMING INCREASINGLY COMMON.

measures fluctuations in your energy field as the stylus is placed at different points, indicating which organs may be out of balance. Homeopathic dilutions of allergens, such as pollen, house dust, dairy produce, feathers or fur, can also be brought into the electronic circuit. An erratic reading is produced when your body is intolerant of a particular substance. The technique can also be used in order to verify which homeopathic remedies your body needs.

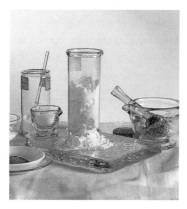

◀ IT IS POSSIBLE TO DESENSITIZE THE BODY USING HOMEOPATHIC REMEDIES OF COMMON ALLERGENS, SUCH AS DUST OR POLLEN.

diagnosis by dowsing

Dowsing is an ancient art that can be used to diagnose energy imbalances and to detect invisible energy pathways. With a little practice, anyone can dowse. All you need is a simple pendulum and an open mind.

PRINCIPLES OF DOWSING

Dowsing is a method of divining or "tapping into" the intelligence of the life force to gain access to information. Holding a pendulum, the dowser will ask a clear, unambiguous "yes/no" question. The pendulum picks up on the energetic vibrations pertaining to the question and then moves in response. The direction of this movement indicates whether the response is positive or negative.

▼ A PENDULUM IS A POPULAR DOWSING TOOL. IT CAN BE MADE FROM METAL, WOOD, POLISHED STONE OR CRYSTAL, BUT IT'S UP TO YOU TO CHOOSE ONE THAT FEELS RIGHT.

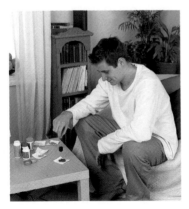

USING DOWSING

Dowsing is extremely useful as a diagnostic technique when you are working with healing energies. For instance, you can dowse to check whether certain foods and vitamins are suitable for you, to detect allergies, to find out which colours, crystals or flower essences are helpful and even to find out where is the best place to live.

You can also dowse when giving healing, to find out where energy is blocked and to check when the energy is flowing again. The key to successful dowsing is asking the right question and remaining objective about the answer that comes back – it's rather like watching for the results of an internet search. Frame your questions clearly and hold the pendulum over the place or article in question. Reassess your findings at regular intervals to stay up-to-date with your changing needs.

TUNING IN

Before you dowse you need to establish the particular pendulum motions that will mean "yes" and "no" for you. Once you are confident and also familiar with the responses, you are ready to start dowsing.

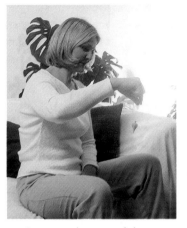

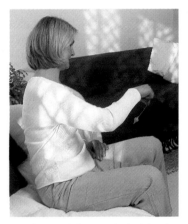

1 Sit upright and hold the pendulum over your lap. Allow it to swing back and forth. This is the "neutral" position.

2 Move the pendulum over your dominant-side knee. State clearly in your mind, "Please show me my 'yes' response." Pay close attention to what the pendulum does as this will be your signal for "yes".

3 Return the pendulum to "neutral", then repeat step 2, moving to your non-dominant side to find the "no" response.

PENDULUM RESPONSES

The diagrams show classic pendulum dowsing responses. Dowsing responses are a very individual and personal thing, however, and you need not worry if yours are not the same as these. What is important is that you are clear which response means "yes", which means "no" and which is "neutral", and then you work with those.

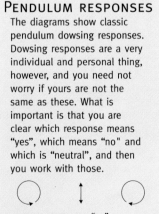

ANTI-CLOCKWISE FOR "NO"
TOWARDS AND AWAY FOR "NEUTRAL"
CLOCKWISE FOR "YES"

diagnosis by applied kinesiology

Applied kinesiology, or muscle testing, is a way of finding and correcting energy imbalances before they become serious health problems. It can also be used to find the underlying causes of long-standing illnesses.

MUSCLE TESTING

In the 1960s, George Goodheart, an American chiropractor, realized that muscles can tell us a great deal about our state of health. He found that the muscles could be strengthened by pressing, and by massaging other, seemingly unrelated, areas of the body. This is because the body is an integral whole, with all its major organs and systems connected by "energy circuits" or meridians. They power the system and link the muscles to different organs.

Excess or blocked energy in these channels can lead to weakness in the corresponding organ and can be detected in the relevant muscle. For example, the quadriceps in the thigh is linked to the small intestine; if you were sensitive to dairy products and drank a glass of milk, then the intolerance would register in the intestine, then in the quadriceps. By testing the strength of various muscles, a kinesiologist can work "backwards" to find out where the underlying problem resides.

▼ KINESIOLOGISTS ALSO USE MASSAGE TECHNIQUES TO BALANCE THE BODY AND TO STRENGTHEN AREAS OF WEAKNESS.

▼ DURING A CONSULTATION YOU WILL BE ASKED ABOUT YOUR MEDICAL HISTORY AND CURRENT MENTAL AND EMOTIONAL STATE.

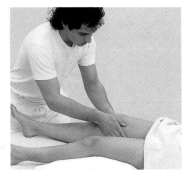

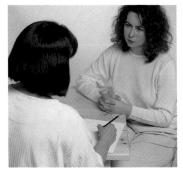

The triangle of health

Kinesiology recognizes that there are three aspects to health – structural (or physical), mental and chemical – and that wellbeing is influenced in all three areas. A kinesiology session involves physical, chemical and/or mental "challenges" during which the patient is asked to resist pressure against an exerted limb. The muscle's energy circuit will "turn off" when an imbalance disrupts a particular pathway.

• Physical challenge: if your health problem is structural, pressure will be applied directly to the bones and muscles to find out where the problem is located.

• Chemical challenge: chemical substances, foods or homeopathic dilutions are placed directly on the tongue or skin, often in a glass phial. These tests are used for allergies.

• Mental challenge: you may be asked to focus on certain thoughts or feelings while the practitioner tests your muscle strength. In fact, many chronic illnesses have a strong emotional component, and you may find out more about the underlying cause of the complaint.

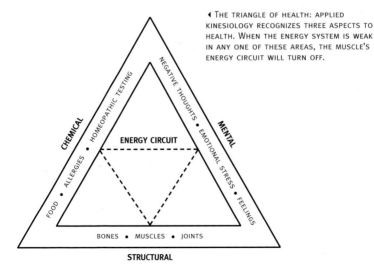

◀ THE TRIANGLE OF HEALTH: APPLIED KINESIOLOGY RECOGNIZES THREE ASPECTS TO HEALTH. WHEN THE ENERGY SYSTEM IS WEAK IN ANY ONE OF THESE AREAS, THE MUSCLE'S ENERGY CIRCUIT WILL TURN OFF.

CHEMICAL

HOMEOPATHIC TESTING

FOOD • ALLERGIES

NEGATIVE THOUGHTS • EMOTIONAL STRESS • FEELINGS

MENTAL

ENERGY CIRCUIT

BONES • MUSCLES • JOINTS

STRUCTURAL

diagnosis by applied kinesiology **21**

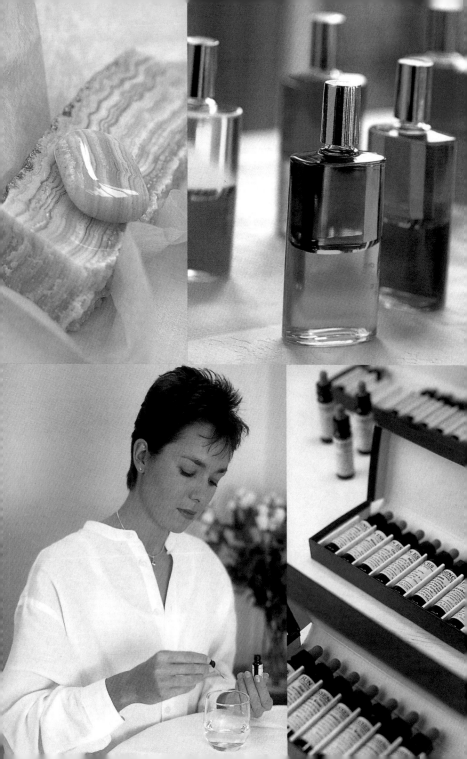

energy therapies

Energy therapies work with subtle vibrations,
attuned to the human energy field, to restore
balance and harmony, and help you return
to physical, mental and emotional health.
The therapies range from taking energy
medicines, such as homeopathy or flower
and gemstone essences, to working with the
healing energies of magnets, water, light,
sound and colour. Many of these techniques
can be safely practised at home, but some,
such as acupuncture and radionics, can only
be carried out by a qualified practitioner.
Always be sure to seek professional advice if
you are uncertain.

homeopathy

 Homeopathy is a system that stimulates the body to heal itself. Homeopathic remedies are prepared from plant, mineral and other extracts, but diluted to such an extent that only the "energy" of the original substance remains.

LIKE CURES LIKE

Homeopathy has been an established system for about 200 years. Discovered by Samuel Hahnemann, a German doctor, it is based on the "law of similars" or the principle that like cures like: the symptoms caused by too much of a substance can also be cured with a small dose of it. For instance, in a patient suffering from insomnia, a homeopath may prescribe the remedy coffea (coffee), which in normal doses would cause sleeplessness in a healthy person.

▼ HOMEOPATHIC REMEDIES ARE PREPARED FROM NUMEROUS DIFFERENT PLANT, ANIMAL AND MINERAL SOURCES. THE ORIGINAL SUBSTANCE IS DILUTED MANY TIMES.

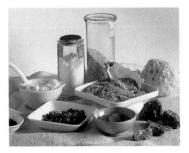

REMEDY PICTURES

Homeopathy is concerned not only with physical symptoms, but also with your mental and emotional state, and remedies are selected on the basis of matching your overall "picture" with a suitable remedy. While two people may suffer from the same illness, they will not necessarily be prescribed the same remedy, as each person is unique. You can use homeopathy to treat yourself for minor acute illnesses, but for chronic conditions you should seek professional advice.

ENERGY MEDICINE

Homeopathic remedies contain no chemical trace of the original substance. They are prepared through dilution and succussion (shaking) to leave only an energy "blueprint". This is then "broadcast" to your energy field, to stimulate the body's powers of healing on the mental, emotional and physical levels.

flower essences

Flower essences are similar to homeopathic remedies. Each essence contains the vibrational pattern of the original plant. They are useful for treating negative mental and emotional states, and for restoring equilibrium.

Flower essences seem to work on the emotional subtle body, with consequent healing effects on the physical body. The Bach flower essences are among the most popular. Dr Edward Bach found that by attuning himself to the subtle vibrations of particular plants, he was able to pick up on their unique characteristics, which could then be utilized for healing.

Bach believed that the vibrational character or spirit of the plant was strongest in its flowers, and that this character could be absorbed as an energy pattern by water, particularly when combined with sunlight. The vibrations will then be absorbed when small amounts of the water are ingested. The drops can be taken directly on the tongue or mixed with a drink of water.

MAKING A FLOWER REMEDY

You can mix your own remedy and make up your own dosing bottles to be taken when needed.

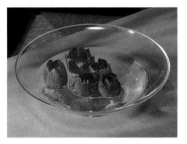

1 Place one to seven blossoms in a bowl for $^1/_2$ litre (1 pint) of remedy. Add water, about two-thirds of the total volume of remedy, and leave in sunlight for two to four hours.

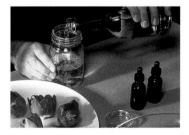

2 Pour the water into a clean glass jar and add half as much vinegar or alcohol, such as brandy or whisky, in order to sterilize and stabilize the remedy. Place the lid on the jar and keep in a cool, dark place. Use as required.

acupuncture

Acupuncture has been practised in China for thousands of years and is one of the oldest systems of healing. It involves inserting fine needles into specific points on the body to regulate the flow of energy through the meridians.

YIN AND YANG

In Chinese thought, the universe is characterized by opposing but complementary energies called "yin" and "yang". Together, they make up "chi" or the vital energy of the life force. Inner harmony is achieved when chi is balanced between these polarities and flows freely through the body, energizing and purifying the organs, tissues and blood. An excess or deficiency in either yin or yang, and/or blocks in the flow of chi, will lead to illness.

CHI AND THE MERIDIANS

The chi is the energy equivalent of the immune system; it supports, nourishes and defends the whole person against disease. Chi runs through the body along energy channels or meridians, which are the equivalent of the arteries and veins of the physical body.

There are 12 main meridians – of which six are yin and six yang – and many minor ones. Together they form an intricate network. Each meridian is named after an organ or function. The yin organs, such as the liver, are "solid", whereas the yang organs, such as the stomach, are "hollow". Along

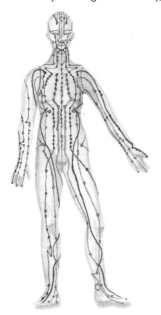

◀ FINE ENERGY CHANNELS, OR MERIDIANS, RUN THROUGH THE BODY, LINKING ITS SYSTEMS AND ORGANS. ACUPUNCTURE IS A TREATMENT THAT TAPS INTO THESE PATHWAYS AT SPECIFIC POINTS.

the meridians are approximately 365 acupuncture points where the chi is concentrated.

TREATMENT

During an acupuncture treatment, extremely fine needles are gently inserted into the skin at the relevant points to stimulate or reduce the flow of chi through the meridian. This may produce a pulling or tugging sensation, but it does not hurt like a normal needle or damage the skin. Needles are usually inserted to a depth of 6–12 mm (¹/₄–¹/₂ in) and left in position for anything from a few seconds to an hour. It is usual for between 6 to 12 needles to be used, at a combination of acupuncture points. It is common to experience a heaviness in the limbs and/or feelings of deep relaxation. If the imbalance is due

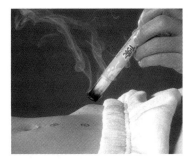

▲ MOXA STICKS ARE OFTEN USED IN AN ACUPUNCTURE TREATMENT TO BALANCE EXCESS YIN (COLD AND DAMP) IN THE BODY.

to a yang deficiency, then the herb moxa (or mugwort) may be burned to generate heat. Dried moxa is rolled into a stick, which is lit and held over the acupuncture point until it becomes too hot.

Acupuncture is a very effective method of pain relief. It has been used in place of anaesthetics during surgery, in dentistry and in childbirth, and is widely used to treat back pain, arthritis and other chronic conditions. Having acupuncture usually leads to an increase in energy, an improved appetite and better sleep, as well as an improved sense of general wellbeing. It should only be carried out by a qualified practitioner.

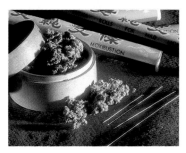

◀ MOXA IS USUALLY DRIED AND THEN ROLLED INTO CIGAR-LIKE STICKS.

Reiki healing

Reiki is a form of spiritual healing that originated in Japan. It works by drawing on "rei-ki" or universal-life energy, which is channelled to areas of need. Giving and receiving Reiki is a gentle and relaxing experience.

CHANNELLING THE POWER OF LOVE

The purpose of Reiki is to work for the "highest good". It connects with the force of unconditional love, which transcends time and space and promotes positive living and compassion for all. To learn Reiki it is usual to go through a special "attunement" with a qualified Reiki master, using ancient and secret symbols to attune the physical and subtle bodies to spiritual energies and opening up a healing channel for them. This channel remains active for life, although the more you use it, the more effective it will be. You can visualize the force as a beam of white light, entering your body and flowing out of your hands when you give healing.

REIKI TREATMENTS

A non-invasive form of healing, Reiki soothes away troubles and traumas in a peaceful way. Certain hand positions are used to dissolve energy blocks and re-balance the body. You can treat yourself with Reiki, as well as others, and you can also use it to treat sick plants and animals and in the environment to guard against negative energy.

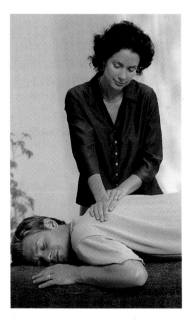

◀ THE PERSON CHANNELLING REIKI IS NEVER DRAINED, AS THE ENERGY FLOWS NOT FROM BUT THROUGH THE HEALER, RATHER LIKE WATER THROUGH A PIPE, AND INTO THE PERSON OR OBJECT BEING HEALED.

A ten-minute Reiki treatment will refresh and energize you and fill you with positive, loving energy.

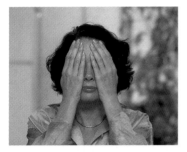

1 Place both hands over your eyes, close them and then relax. This helps to restore strained eyes and clear tension headaches. Move your hands to your temples to help clear an overactive or tired mind.

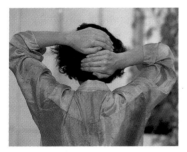

2 Move your hands round to the back of the head and neck area, dispelling tension and refreshing the brain.

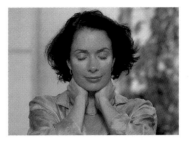

3 Put your hands on either side of your neck. This helps the thyroid gland and the area associated with communication.

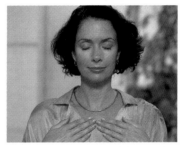

4 Place your hands above the breasts in order to help with lymph drainage and the clearing of toxins. This position may generate some warmth.

5 Finally, move your hands down to the sternum, fingers meeting at the heart chakra. This helps to restore emotional equilibrium. Finish with your hands below the navel to centre yourself.

crystals and gems

Crystals and gemstones have always been prized for their magical and therapeutic qualities. These treasures from the earth are able to store, magnify and transform energy, and have unique properties that can be used in healing.

STABILITY AND BALANCE

The properties of crystals derive from their unique orderliness and the stability of their atomic structure, which is not upset by outside forces such as heat or pressure. This may explain why they can work on imbalances in our subtle energy system. Amethyst balances the energy bodies, clear quartz strengthens and cleanses, and rose quartz is helpful for releasing emotional blocks.

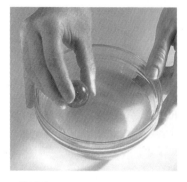

▲ CLEANSE YOUR CRYSTAL BY PLACING IT IN A BOWL OF SALT WATER. THE SALT WILL CLEAR ANY NEGATIVE VIBRATIONS.

PREPARING CRYSTALS FOR HEALING

Because crystals hold energy, it is important that they are always thoroughly cleansed before you use them for healing. You may detect negative vibrations in a stone by a feeling of heaviness or unpleasantness when you handle it. To clean hard stones, place them in a bowl of salt water and leave overnight. Bury softer stones in a bowl of dry sea salt and leave for 24 hours.

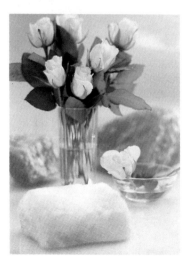

◄ ROSE QUARTZ HAS A CALMING EFFECT AND CAN HELP TO RELEASE EMOTIONS.

A simple way of using crystals in healing is the hand-held method. A quartz crystal will direct the flow of energy either towards or away from the body, depending on which way the point is facing. Hold this in your dominant-side hand; this is the side that "gives out" energy. The opposite hand is your "absorbing" or "receiving" hand. You can select a stone depending on which healing energies you want to work with.

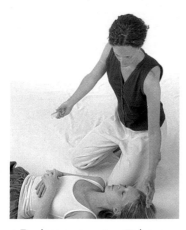

1 To clear away unwanted energy and aid relaxation, hold your "receiving" hand with its stone close to your partner, with the quartz crystal in your "directing" hand pointing downwards. This allows the energy to drain into the earth. Put the "receiving" hand and its stone on areas of the body which seem tense and tight.

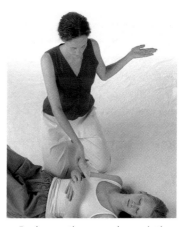

2 Recharge the aura by pointing the "directing" hand and crystal towards the body. Hold the "receiving" hand and stone upwards and visualize energy flowing through you into the newly cleansed area.

CRYSTAL ENERGIES

amethyst: calming, balancing; useful in meditation
clear quartz: strengthens, cleanses and purifies; rebalances energy
rose quartz: releases emotions; promotes love and calm

moon medicine

The moon's phases are associated with important healing energies. Moon medicine combines the power of crystals with the light of a new, full or waning moon, which can empower medicines with healing and calming vibrations.

PHASES OF THE MOON

Timing is very important in moon medicine. The new moon is for health, vitality and regeneration; the full moon for fertility and empowerment; the waning phase is the time when symptoms and ailments may be banished.

CRYSTALS OF THE MOON

Traditionally, all white, clear or watery bright stones are associated with the waxing and full moon, or "bright moontime". Black, dark or cloudy stones are used at the time of the waning moon, or "dark moontime".

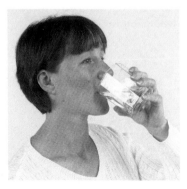

BRIGHT MOONTIME CRYSTALS

Any smooth round white stone as well as the following:

• Moonstone: to balance the hormonal cycle; calm emotions, especially over parenting issues
• Aquamarine: to aid dreams and access to divine guidance
• Pearl: to balance emotions and hormones, increase confidence
• Clear quartz: to enhance and direct the moon's rays in healing

DARK MOONTIME CRYSTALS

Any smooth, circular black stone as well as the following:

• Jet: to calm the subtle bodies, clear the head, lift depression
• Smoky quartz: to re-balance, heal and clear negativity
• Obsidian: to find the cause of energy imbalance
• Black tourmaline: to help physical problems to do with the bones and muscles

◀ DRINKING A CRYSTAL INFUSION EMPOW-
ERED WITH THE MOON'S HEALING ENERGIES
WILL BRING A LITTLE MAGIC INTO YOUR LIFE.

MAKING A CRYSTAL INFUSION

You need to make sure the moon is in the correct phase of its cycle before you begin. This may mean waiting for a while, but will ensure your medicine contains the most appropriate vibrations.

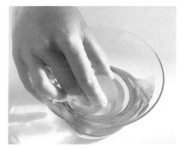

1 To make a crystal or gemstone infusion, select the appropriate crystal. Ensure that it has been cleansed of negative energies in salt water. Hold the stone and visualize the power of the moon infusing it with the healing powers you wish to work with.

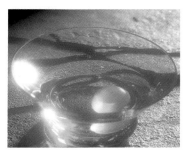

2 Place the stone in a clear glass bowl and cover with spring water. Leave the bowl in the moonlight for several hours or, if possible, overnight. If the weather is calm, then you can place the bowl outside; alternatively, leave it indoors, perhaps in a window or conservatory (sun room), for example, where the moonlight will fall directly on to it. You might also like to use a circle of nightlights to symbolize the light of the moon, but remember not to leave them burning unattended.

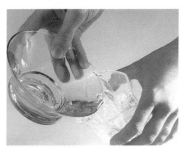

3 Carefully remove the crystal with a pair of tongs, being careful not to touch the water with your hands. Pour the infusion into a glass. Sip the water slowly and, as you drink it, feel the power of the moon's healing rays gently infusing your body, bringing healing peace and harmony.

meditation

Meditation is a state of altered awareness and deep relaxation. It helps to dissolve energy blocks and restore balance and harmony. A 10–15 minute meditation can be as beneficial as several hours of deep sleep.

BALANCING OPPOSITES

The brain has two hemispheres which are responsible for different functions. The dominant left side deals with rational thought, action, speech and logic. The right side is associated with intuition, creativity and emotional responses. Meditation helps to bring the two sides into a state of balance, where neither is holding sway at the expense of the other.

▼ MEDITATION IS A TIME TO SIT, RELAX AND DO NOTHING. IT CAN BALANCE OUR ENERGIES AND BRING HEALING ON MANY LEVELS.

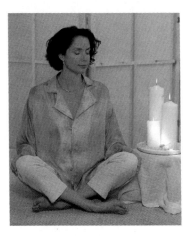

BRAIN WAVES

During meditation, the brain produces a relaxed alpha wave pattern, similar – yet of greater intensity – to that produced during deep sleep. In alpha state, the body is quiet and receptive, restoring us on many levels, physical, mental and emotional.

GOLDEN LIGHT MEDITATION

Sit in a relaxed position, close your eyes and focus on your breathing. As you breathe in, imagine a stream of golden healing light entering your body. Hold the breath for a count of three, and imagine the light circulating through your whole system, passing through the chakras, meridians and all your physical organs. As you breathe out, imagine the darkness of sickness or negativity leaving you, dissolving into light. Repeat this cycle for 10–15 minutes. At the end of the meditation you should feel refreshed and energized.

light therapy

Light plays an important role in psychological and physical health, affecting our moods and immune system. Light therapy simulates natural daylight to treat a range of conditions, including skin problems and depression.

THE POWER OF LIGHT

Daylight is involved with the production of vitamin D, and sunlight also regulates the body's biological clock, affecting sleep patterns, appetite, temperature, sex drive and the production of hormones, including serotonin, the "happy hormone". Our biological clock is designed to be in tune with the natural rhythm of day and night, and seasonal change. Night work, long distance travel and extended periods of time indoors play havoc with our body chemistry, and light deprivation can lead to an impaired functioning of the immune system and depression.

TREATING DEPRESSION

Reduced daylight can cause severe depression. This is now officially recognized as a medical condition and referred to as SAD (seasonal affective disorder). It is often treated with light therapy.

TREATMENT

Light therapy involves lying under a fluorescent full-spectrum, or bright, white light. This has the same effect as daylight, but does not contain the harmful UV rays. Daylight averages about 5,000 lux, whereas normal artificial light averages between 500–1,000. At least 2,500 lux are needed for a therapeutic effect. Professional supervision is recommended.

▼ SOAKING UP THE SUN IS GOOD IN SMALL DOSES. SUNLIGHT CAN LIFT DEPRESSION AND HELP WITH MANY SKIN PROBLEMS.

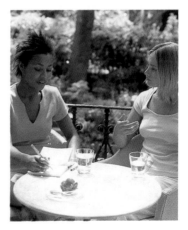

colour vibrations

Each band of energy in the colour spectrum vibrates at a frequency that corresponds with one of the body's organs and energy systems. Colour therapy uses light of the appropriate colour to restore equilibrium in the body.

The psychology of colour

Instinctively we know that colours affect us in different ways. We speak of feeling blue, being in a black mood, being green with envy or red with anger. Every day and in countless ways we are influenced by the distinctive energy vibrations that each colour possesses, whether it is through the colour of our clothes, the food we eat, the rooms we live in or the scenery of the world outside. Colour is intrinsic to life.

▼ Green is the colour of fresh growth and natural harmony. It soothes shock and relieves fatigue.

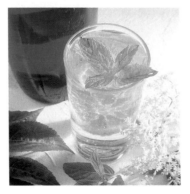

Tuning into colour

It is not necessary to be able to see to have a sense of colour. Many blind people have, in fact, developed their sensitivity to the subtle vibrational energies of different colours in ways that we do not fully understand. For instance, the Aura-Soma colour system was developed in the 1980s by a British woman, Vicky Wall, after she lost her sight. The system uses colour essences in different combinations, which may be used in the bath or on the skin, to help balance emotional, spiritual and psychological states.

Choosing colours

Use the colour vibration chart to help you select the colour that you feel is the most appropriate for you. If you are not sure which colour you need, use your intuition to choose the one that most attracts you. You can use dowsing with a pendulum to check your selection.

Colour vibrations
Choose colours according to your healing need or preference

colour	properties	healing uses
red	stimulating, energizing	low energy, sexual problems, blood disorders, lack of confidence
orange	cheering, enlivening	depression, mental disorders, asthma, rheumatism
yellow	inspiring, helping mental clarity and detachment	detoxifying, hormonal problems (menopause, menstrual difficulties)
green	fresh, vibrant, harmonious, idealistic	antiseptic, balancing, tonic, good for shock and fatigue, soothes headaches
blue	soothing, calming, promoting truth and inner reflection	insomnia, nervous disorders, throat problems, general healing
indigo	transforming, purifying	painkiller, sinus problems, migraine, eczema, inflammations, chest complaints, insomnia
violet/ purple	regal, dignifying	love of self, self-respect, psychological disorders and problems with the scalp (use sparingly, as purple is a "heavy" colour)
magenta	letting go	emotional hurts and upsets, accepting life's problems
black	absorbing, secretive	for when you need to hide (such as when grieving), or alternatively to convey an impression of power and control; self-discipline
white	reflecting, purity, innocence	a tonic; replaces all colours
gold	divine power, purity, the sun	depression and low energy, digestive disturbances, rheumatism, scars
silver	cosmic intelligence, the moon	hormonal and emotional balance, calms the nerves, for recovering equilibrium

healing with colour

There are countless ways of harnessing the vibration of colour for health and wellbeing. You can wear it, use it in your surroundings, make colour infusions, eat different coloured food, or even bathe in coloured light.

COLOUR INFUSIONS

It is easy to make your own colour essences. Use coloured stones, coloured fabric or any other colourfast item, and soak your "colour" in a bowl of mineral water. Leave the bowl in sunlight for several hours. Pour the water into a glass and then drink the infusion. Always make sure the coloured item you are using is clean before you soak it.

▼ WE CAN BENEFIT FROM THE HEALING VIBRATIONS OF COLOUR USING FABRIC AND CLOTHING. BLUE IS A GOOD GENERAL HEALER.

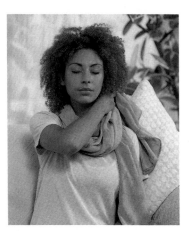

MOOD FOODS

Different coloured foods can heal and stimulate health. Red, orange and yellow foods are hot and stimulating. Yellow foods can help with weight loss, and red foods restore energy. Green balances and detoxifies, and is a tonic for the system. Blue, indigo and purple are soothing; blue curbs activity so is useful when you are trying to put on weight.

▼ USE THE COLOURS OF YOUR FOOD TO REJUVENATE AND BALANCE THE MIND-BODY SYSTEM. FRESH ORGANIC FOODS ARE BEST.

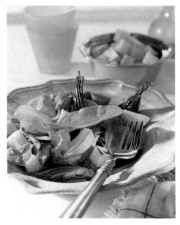

CHROMOTHERAPY

Healing with colour involves shining coloured light on to the body to relieve physical, mental and emotional problems. You can use it at home or perhaps seek professional guidance for more complicated problems. The principle is very simple. Using different coloured gels or slides in front of high-powered lamps, you can bathe the body with any colour needed for healing. A quartz-tipped "crystal flashlight", about the size of a marker pen, can also be used to direct the coloured light on to specific points on the body, a technique that is sometimes known as "colour puncture".

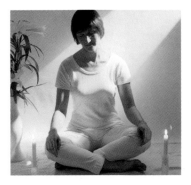

▲ BATHE YOURSELF IN THE GREEN VIBRATION TO ENCOURAGE POSITIVE THOUGHTS AND BRING CREATIVITY.

TREATMENT

The main colour choice is often followed by its complementary opposite. For instance, if you are being treated with green, this may be followed by magenta to ensure a healthy balance in the body. Treatment sessions normally last for up to an hour and are then repeated over several weeks.

At home you can use a free-standing spotlight. Place a coloured gel over the spotlight, making sure it is not touching the hot bulb. Turn off any other lights and bathe in the coloured light, taking in the healing vibrations of your chosen colour.

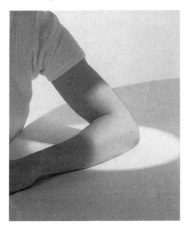

◀ ORANGE LIGHT DIRECTED ON TO A STIFF JOINT CAN HELP TO RELEASE THE LIGAMENTS.

water therapies

Water is the elixir of life. It covers more than two-thirds of the earth's surface and our bodies are largely made from water. There are many ways of using water's cleansing and rejuvenating powers to increase health and vitality.

DETOX TREATMENTS

Hydrotherapy is based on improving elimination of waste products, and there are simple treatments you can build into your daily routine. Drinking plenty of water will help your body flush out toxins and increase energy levels. Sweating expels impurities through the skin: vigorous exercise, saunas or steam baths are ideal. Take plenty of showers to wash away the toxins.

HOT AND COLD

Cold water has a stimulating effect, constricting the blood vessels and inhibiting biochemical reactions that cause inflammation. It helps to energize and cleanse the organs and subtle energy system. Taking a cold shower seals the body's aura, stopping energy from leaking out.

Warm or hot water dilates the blood vessels, increasing the flow of blood to the skin and reducing

▼ GET INTO THE WATER HABIT. DRINKING BETWEEN 6 AND 8 GLASSES A DAY WILL HELP TO KEEP YOUR ENERGY LEVELS HIGH.

▼ RAW FRUIT AND VEGETABLES HAVE A HIGH WATER CONTENT. INCLUDE PLENTY IN YOUR DIET TO HELP YOUR BODY DETOX.

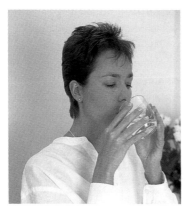

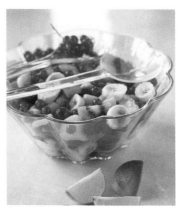

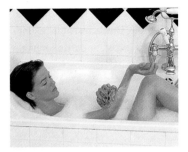

◄ WATER IS A POWERFUL CLEANSER. IT NOT ONLY CLEANS THE PHYSICAL BODY, BUT ALSO REMOVES PSYCHIC DIRT HELD IN THE AURA.

blood pressure. Warm water has a relaxing effect and can help to ease psychological and muscular tension by "drawing things" to the surface to be released.

FLOTATION THERAPY

Combining the benefits of water with meditation, flotation therapy involves "floating" in warm water in an environment that is free from external stimuli. Salts and minerals are dissolved in the water to enable the body to float without any effort.

Sessions normally last from 1 to 1½ hours and take place in a sound- and light-proof tank or bath a little larger than the body. The water is maintained at skin temperature (34.2°C/93.5°F) and you can switch on a light or open the tank at any time. The effect is profoundly relaxing for both body and mind. The brain releases endorphins (the body's natural painkillers) and many people experience feelings of euphoria. Flotation therapy has a deep-cleansing and balancing effect on the subtle bodies and is particularly useful for treating stress and anxiety. It also helps to relieve hypertension (high blood pressure), tension headaches, back pain and muscle fatigue, and is a good immunity booster.

HYDRATION

Some experts believe that dehydration underlies many health problems. Water helps to flush out toxins and keep the cells and organs healthy. Drinking 2–3 litres (3½–5½ pints) of water a day, cutting down on tea, coffee and alcohol – all of which are dehydrating – and eating more raw food (which has a high water content) is a good way to gain vitality. At first you may feel more tired, but after a few weeks you will notice that your energy levels increase and your skin will start to look fresher and clearer.

chakra balancing

The seven chakras are the gateways by which the vital force enters and leaves the body. These invisible energy centres govern the major glands in the endocrine system and influence our health at all levels.

ENERGY TRANSFORMERS

The chakras are located along a central energy channel, which corresponds to the spinal cord, from the base of the spine to the head. They are often imagined as vibrantly coloured, many-petalled lotus flowers. Each one resonates with a particular vibrational frequency, which descends from the highest at the top of the head, to the lowest at the base of the spine, transforming and balancing the body's energy as it moves through the system.

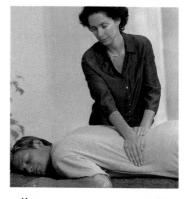

▲ MANY COMMON STRESS-RELATED HEALTH PROBLEMS ARE RELATED TO IMBALANCE IN THE THIRD CHAKRA. PLACE YOUR HANDS ON EITHER SIDE OF THE RIBCAGE NEAR THE KIDNEYS AND ALLOW THE HEALING ENERGY TO RECHARGE THIS AREA.

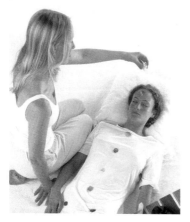

BALANCING THE CHAKRAS

Chakras operate on many levels, nourishing every part of our bodies with life-force energy. They are connected to each other and to our physical cellular structure by threads of subtle energy, or "nadis", similar to the meridians of Chinese acupuncture. They can be thrown out of balance by many

◀ BALANCE THE CHAKRAS WITH GEMSTONES OF THE RELEVANT COLOUR ON EACH CHAKRA.

things, including poor diet, lack of sleep and exercise, high stress levels, pharmaceutical medicines and negative influences, such as electrical energy fields, geopathic stress and pollution.

Treatment

There are many ways to balance the chakras. For instance, you could work with colour therapy and gemstones, placing the appropriate coloured stone on each of the chakra points as you lie on the floor. Or you could use the healing properties of sound by intoning the mantra (healing sound) relevant to each energy centre, beginning from the base and ascending to the crown, and down again.

Alternatively, you can use Reiki and work with your hands, channelling healing energy into all the relevant chakra points, working up the front of the body, or down the spine. To diagnose which chakras are out of balance, you can use your pendulum and dowse over them; you can also use dowsing after the treatment in order to check that the imbalance has been corrected.

CHAKRA PROPERTIES
Each chakra corresponds to a colour and sound, and governs distinct areas

1st Root: red (mantra: "lam") gonads or ovaries, skeleton, large intestine and lower body; physical survival, energy distribution, practicality

2nd Sacral: orange (mantra: "vam") bladder, circulation; sexuality, creativity, feelings, emotions and pleasure

3rd Solar plexus: yellow (mantra: "ram") adrenal glands, spleen, pancreas, stomach; identity, confidence, personal power, desires

4th Heart: green (mantra: "yam") thymus gland, immune system, lungs; relationships, personal development, compassion, self-acceptance

5th Throat: blue (mantra: "ham") thyroid, lymphatic, immune and neurological systems; self-expression, communication, trust

6th Brow/"third eye": indigo (mantra: "om") pituitary gland, central nervous system; understanding, perception, intuition, insight, spiritual knowing, psychic abilities

7th Crown: violet (silence) pineal gland, ancient mammalian brain; openness, connection to higher energies, self-realization

feng shui

Dating back more than 1000 years, the Chinese art of feng shui is concerned with environmental influences on health and wellbeing. It offers practical suggestions of ways to balance the invisible energies in our surroundings.

CHI PATHS

According to ancient Chinese philosophy, our destiny is shaped by environmental forces, or the unseen energies that swirl all around us. Just as energy moves through the human body along the meridians, so it moves throughout the world around us, travelling along invisible energy pathways or "chi paths". Similarly, the energy in the environment is characterized in terms of the opposition between yin and yang. For instance, quiet and stillness

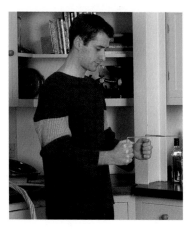

are yin, noise and activity are yang. Round shapes, such as curves or circles, soft drapes and dark, absorbing colours enhance yin energy, whereas angular shapes and patterns, straight hangings and bright reflecting colours enhance yang energy.

BALANCING CHI

The purpose of feng shui is to create an environment in which chi flows smoothly and an even balance between yin and yang is maintained. This helps to create the right conditions for growth – no matter whether you are trying to create a happy home life, a successful business or a beautiful garden. Chi that is out of balance creates stagnant or excess energy pools, which in turn creates disharmony and disruption, as well as possible sickness and exhaustion.

◀ FOR DETECTING CHI PATHS, L-SHAPED METAL RODS ARE EASIER TO WORK WITH THAN A PENDULUM. KEEP HIGH-USE AREAS ENERGETICALLY CLEAR AND WELL BALANCED.

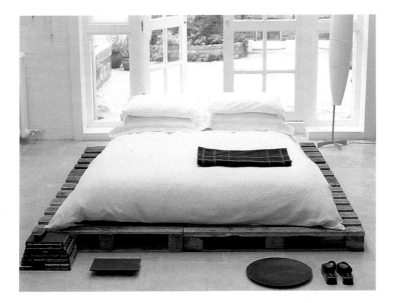

WORKING WITH FENG SHUI

Landscapes, buildings, rooms and everything in them vibrate with energy. Human beings function best when they are in the same range of vibrations as the earth. Using natural materials in your home will help to promote positive chi. Synthetic materials, chemicals, microwave ovens and electrical equipment all create negative chi. To help balance the effects of this chi, use crystals and/or plants near computers and television sets, and limit the time you spend using them.

▲ KEEPING YOUR SURROUNDINGS CLEAN AND CLUTTER-FREE HELPS CHI TO FLOW SMOOTHLY AND PROMOTES A CALM ATMOSPHERE.

DETECTING CHI PATHS

If you suffer from ill health or chronic tiredness, or your plans continually go awry, you may be exposed to negative chi paths. You can dowse to find the chi paths in your home and to indicate where chi is blocked or stagnant. Notice the health of any plants on the path and whether it runs under beds or chairs. It is best not to sleep or spend long periods directly in chi paths.

healing sounds

Sound therapy is one of the oldest and most profound forms of energy healing. From the simple repetition of mystical words to complex rhythms and structures, sound waves can alter our mood and enhance wellbeing.

A UNIVERSE OF SOUNDS

Sound is our first experience of life. In the womb, a baby becomes familiar with the mother's heartbeat and voice. We feel most at ease with naturally occurring sound frequencies, such as the human voice, a running stream, birdsong, or rustling leaves. Constant exposure to discordant noises and high levels of background noise, such as from traffic, undermines the sensitivity

▾ THE POWERFUL HEALING VIBRATIONS OF A GONG CAN HELP "CLEAR THE AIR" OF NEGATIVE ENERGIES.

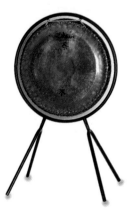

MANTRA

A mantra is a sacred sound that is used to "tune" the body's vibrational field and to raise levels of consciousness. In the Hindu tradition, the "om" mantra is believed to be the original sound from which the universe was born.

of our hearing and is a source of stress. Sound pollution weakens the immune system and has been linked to anxiety and depression.

VIBRATIONAL FIELDS

We pick up on sound waves not only through our ears, but also through our vibrational energy field. The subtle bodies, the chakras, and the physical body all vibrate at particular frequencies. When these vibrations are thrown out of balance, we are literally "out of tune", and become unwell. Sound therapy uses specific sound waves to retune these vibrations and restore harmony.

Using the voice

The voice is an almost unlimited source of healing energy. Simple ways to work with it include chanting, toning and singing. Tones are pure sounds held on a single note, such as "aaaaa..." or "uuuuu...". Practised regularly, toning has a powerful effect on the body's cells and can raise energy levels, help to release emotional trauma and promote mental clarity. It can be combined with chanting, which involves the repetition of a mantra or short phrase. Chanting is one of the oldest singing techniques and has its roots in spiritual traditions.

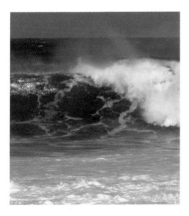

▼ The rhythmic sound of waves as they crash on the shore can have a calming effect on the spirit.

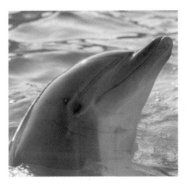

▲ Many people experience a sense of euphoria when they hear the high frequency sounds of dolphins.

Music

Listening to music that is at the same frequency as alpha and theta brainwave patterns can promote relaxation and insight. Certain instruments, such as bells and gongs, generate particularly powerful healing sounds and their vibrations can be used to "clear the air" of negative energies.

Benefits

Healing sounds can dissolve tension, regulate heart rate and breathing, increase mental clarity and raise consciousness. Some high frequency sounds encourage the release of endorphins, and can produce feelings of bliss and euphoria.

magnetotherapy

Magnets have been widely used in healing for thousands of years. A magnet generates an electromagnetic field (EMF) that can be used to influence the body's natural energy circuits to treat many common complaints.

USING MAGNETS

Magnets have the ability to speed up the flow of liquids and to prevent the clogging of channels. This gives them many benefits. For instance, they can be fitted to water pipes to reduce the build-up of scale; the magnets create a magnetic field that keeps the positively charged calcium ions (the ones that cause the scale) in suspension and away from the inner walls of the pipe.

▼ PLACING MAGNETS AT STRATEGIC POINTS ON THE BODY CAN RELIEVE MENSTRUAL PAIN AND OTHER EVERYDAY AILMENTS.

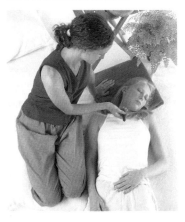

MAGNET THERAPY

Magnets can improve the flow of blood through the veins. They can help to clear blocked arteries, improve oxygen supply to the cells, stimulate the metabolism, and help with the elimination of waste. There is growing evidence that they ease muscle and joint pain and reduce inflammation. Magnets can be used to treat a variety of conditions, including arthritis, respiratory disorders, menstrual problems, headaches and insomnia.

Magnetic healthcare products include straps and wristbands, mattresses, car seat covers and shoe insoles, as well as special devices to fit to plumbing and heating systems. The magnet is worn or placed either at the site of pain, over lymph nodes (to encourage the drainage of toxins), or at specific acupuncture points. Many wearers report increased energy levels, improved mental clarity and general wellbeing.

radionics

Radionics is a method of distant healing that uses specially designed instruments to analyse and treat energy imbalances. It was pioneered in the 1920s by Dr Albert Abrams, an American neurologist.

THE WITNESS

During the course of his work, Abrams devised a special machine, which became known as "the black box", with which to read the pattern of his patients' energy fields. This pattern is held in every cell of the body and can be witnessed in any of its parts, such as a drop of blood, a nail clipping or a lock of hair. Provided any small part can be given to the radionics practitioner as a "witness", it is not necessary for the patient to be present for diagnosis and treatment.

TREATMENT

You will be asked to complete a health-check questionnaire and send a hair or blood sample to the practitioner, to act as the witness, and to provide an "energetic link" between you. The witness is then placed on a black box and readings are taken to indicate your physical, mental and emotional state, your energy flow,

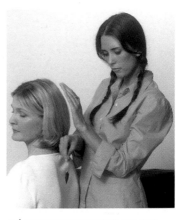

▲ A RADIONICS PRACTITIONER MAY ALSO USE DOWSING TO VERIFY HIS OR HER DIAGNOSIS AND TREATMENT PLAN.

any indications of major diseases and the cause of any existing health problem. Once a diagnosis has been made, the black box is used to "broadcast" healing energy to you. Some practitioners may also suggest homeopathic or Bach flower remedies, or colour therapy. Radionics aims to improve general health and wellbeing and is particularly helpful for diagnosing and treating allergies.

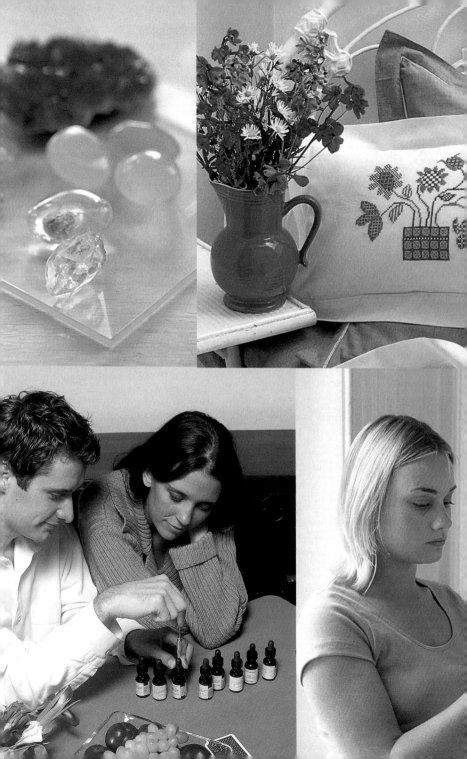

treatments for common ailments

Many everyday health problems can be helped with energy therapies. The following pages discuss ailments ranging from colds and flu to arthritis and chronic fatigue syndrome. Stress, emotional problems and food sensitivities are also included.

Advice is given on which therapies are particularly suited to each condition, with specific treatments that can be safely self-administered at home. But always be sure to seek professional help for long-standing chronic complaints or if you are uncertain. And remember, your energy is your most precious commodity: use it wisely.

stress

A certain amount of stress is healthy, providing challenge and stimulation, but when faced with too much pressure the body responds by working harder until finally we get sick. Many common health problems are stress-related.

Financial pressures, problems in relationships, bereavement or divorce, moving house, getting married, noise and traffic are all common "stressors" that most of us cannot avoid.

Meditation, calming colours and healing sounds can all help to reduce stress levels. Kinesiology has specific techniques to help with the release of emotional stress, and will also check for any nutritional deficiencies. Dowse to check you are getting enough vitamin B, which is used up more quickly when you are under stress.

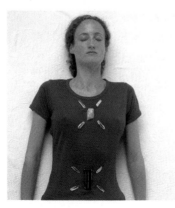

TREATMENT FOR SHOCK

Use a crystal layout after a shock to help release stress and prevent the trauma from seeping deeply into your energy system. Put a rose quartz stone at your heart centre, with four clear quartz points facing outwards around it, to release emotional tension. Put a tiger's eye at the sacral chakra with another four quartz points, to stabilize and ground the energy.

HOMEOPATHIC REMEDIES

These work to boost your "vital force" and are prescribed on an individual basis. However, some may be useful in acute situations:
• Ignatia 6c: soothes grief and disappointment
• Nux vomica 6c: helps with stress from overwork and irritability
• Sepia 6c: when you feel unable to cope, weepy and irritable
• Phos ac 6c: for stress due to grief or bad news

◀ USE THIS CRYSTAL LAYOUT TO RELIEVE THE STRESS OF A SHOCK OR ACCIDENT.

depression

Most people experience mood swings as well as the highs and lows of life. However, persistent worries, fears and tensions create energy blocks and we can get stuck on a "low" if we do not find a way to release the energy.

There are many triggers to negative mood states, including worries related to your state of health, finances, children or relationship problems. Physical illness or hormonal changes, such as those of menstruation, childbirth and menopause, may also be involved.

To encourage a more optimistic mood, use cheerful and enlivening colours, such as yellow or orange, with a touch of pink if you are feeling emotionally upset.

▾ WHEN YOUR SPIRITS ARE LOW, FLOWER REMEDIES CAN HELP RESTORE WELLBEING.

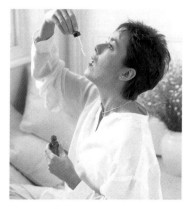

Avoid wearing black, grey and dark colours, and over-exposing yourself to "negative vibes" in the environment: this can include reading too much distressing news. Plenty of exposure to natural light, especially sunshine, is very helpful.

BACH FLOWERS
There are several Bach flower remedies that can help with depression. Select the one that most closely matches how you feel.
- Gorse: hopelessness and despair due to a setback
- Sweet chestnut: utter dejection and bleak outlook
- Mustard: gloom descends like a black cloud for no obvious reason
- Willow: introspective, pessimistic; self-pitying
- Honeysuckle: dwelling on the past, lack of interest in the present

MUSTARD   HONEYSUCKLE

restful sleep

Most adults need seven to eight hours' sleep a night, when the body's systems shut down to permit healing and renewal. Lack of sleep is a common problem that is very debilitating, physically, mentally and emotionally.

Difficulties in getting to sleep, or a broken sleep pattern, may be caused by a variety of problems, including stress and worry, physical pain, illness, lack of exercise, changes in body-clock rhythms (due to jet lag or shift work, for instance), as well as too much caffeine, alcohol or nicotine.

There are many steps you can take to ensure a good night's sleep. Avoid over-stimulating your energy system in the evening and keep the energy pathways in the bedroom clear. Keep electrical equipment away from the bed, and put items like computers and television sets in another room. Make sure the evening is a time when you unwind and let go of the worries of the day. Practising meditation or taking a relaxing bath before bed usually helps.

SLEEP CRYSTALS

Tuning into the subtle vibrations of crystals can also help with sleep problems. Holding the appropriate stone can help to quieten you so that you can relax and fall asleep.

- Chrysoprase: promotes peaceful, healing sleep
- Amethyst, rose quartz or citrine: help when sleeplessness is caused by tension and worry
- Smoky quartz or tourmaline: calm sleep disturbances related to fear, or nightmares. Place the stone at the foot of the bed.

▼ DEEP AND PEACEFUL SLEEP IS ONE OF NATURE'S BEST ENERGY BOOSTERS.

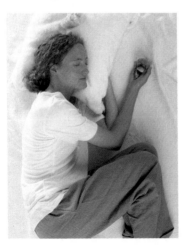

headaches and migraine

Most "everyday" headaches are caused by stress and tension. They can range from a dull throbbing to an intense stabbing pain. Migraines are even more disabling, and are often accompanied by nausea and vomiting.

Headaches can be triggered by a variety of factors, including toxic overload (from prescription drugs, caffeine, alcohol, or junk food), dehydration, low blood sugar, food intolerance, eyestrain, sinusitis, weather conditions and hormonal swings. Migraine triggers may include foodstuffs, such as red wine, chocolate or cheese, and attacks are exacerbated by stress.

Water is one of the best first-aid treatments for headaches and migraine, so drink a glass or two

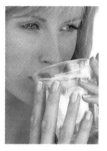

◀ IF YOU FEEL A HEADACHE COMING ON, TRY DRINKING A GLASS OR TWO OF MINERAL WATER. YOU MAY FIND THAT THE HEADACHE JUST DISAPPEARS OR IS AT LEAST LESS PAINFUL.

at the first sign of pain. Splashing your face with water and lying down at the onset of a migraine is also helpful. Tension headaches may be relieved by a bath, sauna or steam bath. Alternating hot and cold will improve circulation.

The colour green is restful on the eyes and may help you to relax, while amethysts can ease tension headaches. For pain relief, press between the thumb and forefinger of each hand, or press your thumbs into the hollow areas at the base of the skull on either side of the spine, and tilt your head back for a few moments, breathing deeply.

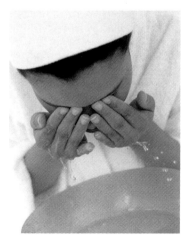

◀ RELIEVE TENSION HEADACHES BY SPLASHING COOL WATER OVER YOUR FACE.

colds and flu

Catching a cold or flu is a sign that your energy levels are depleted and your body's defences are weakened. Colds are often linked with seasonal changes in weather patterns, when the body needs extra support.

In the early "sore throat" stages of a cold, drink hot lemon and honey and eat light meals. In the later stages, eating raw foods and drinking fresh fruit and vegetable juices will have a cleansing and energy-boosting effect, and can help with clearing mucus. Avoid tea, coffee, sugar and dairy products. Resting and giving your body a chance to recover is also essential; carrying on regardless will drain your energy further and, in the long run, may mean that it takes even longer to get better.

▼ RED ONION IS USED TO MAKE THE HOMEOPATHIC REMEDY ALLIUM CEPA. THIS IS INDICATED FOR COLDS WITH PROFUSE SNEEZING AND "CRYING" EYES.

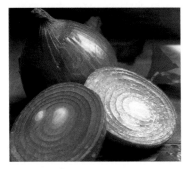

COLOUR TREATMENTS

To ease a sore throat, wrap a blue or green scarf around your neck to bring healing energy to your throat chakra. Alternatively, drink blue or green colour infusions.

HOMEOPATHY CURES

There are several homeopathic remedies for colds and flu.
• Allium cepa 6c: head colds characterized by sneezing
• Ferrum phos 6c: cold that comes on slowly, with a red swollen throat
• Nux vomica 6c: irritability, feeling chilly, watery eyes
• Kali bich 6c: blocked sinuses with yellow-green mucus
• Aconite 6c: sudden onset of flu, often at night, with chill and high fever
• Belladonna 6c: sudden onset of flu, with headache, fever
• Gelsemium 6c: "traditional" flu, with shivers, shakes, aching muscles, debility

FERRUM PHOS   KALI BICH

chronic fatigue syndrome

Chronic fatigue is an extremely disabling condition for which there is no conventional medical treatment. It can be a symptom of a number of conditions, such as depression or anaemia, or may follow a viral infection, such as flu.

CFS is a complicated condition. Its symptoms are a sign that your energy is severely depleted and out of balance. This means that you need to be particularly wary of "energy drainers" and cultivate things that give you energy.

Start by assessing your diet and lifestyle. Find out if you have any food intolerances or allergies; kinesiology, Vega testing, dowsing and radionics can all be used to check for this. Then, consider the impact that electromagnetic energy fields may be having on your health. Is your home or workplace an energy haven or is it draining you? Metal conducts electricity, so don't position a bed near a radiator, or sleep in a brass bed next to a power point. Protect yourself from the electric fields of domestic appliances and make sure your computer screen has low-level radiation. Work with feng

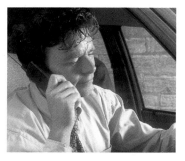

▲ TRY TO AVOID PROLONGED PERIODS WHEN YOU ARE EXPOSED TO STRESS AS THIS WILL DEPLETE YOUR ENERGY LEVELS.

shui to keep energy pathways clear, and use colours that enhance energy: purples and blues to boost the immune system, greens to lift depression, and yellows to promote a positive outlook.

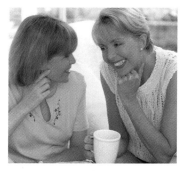

▶ SPENDING TIME WITH FRIENDS NOURISHES THE MENTAL AND EMOTIONAL BODIES AND CAN HELP TO TRIGGER THE BODY'S SELF-HEALING MECHANISMS.

arthritis

There are two types of arthritis. Osteoarthritis is the more common and is marked by degeneration in the cartilage that protects the joints; in rheumatoid arthritis the joints become inflamed and painfully swollen.

According to the World Health Organization, acupuncture is an effective treatment for arthritis and it is increasingly recommended by conventional medicine. Regular acupuncture treatments can help to ease joint pain, stiffness and inflammation, and restore a greater range of movement to the joints.

Water treatments can also be effective; cold compresses can help to relieve pain and swelling, or alternate hot and cold will help to boost the circulation and ease stiffness. Check your diet using kinesiology, dowsing or Vega testing and make sure you are getting enough of the foods, vitamins and minerals that your body needs. Cut down on the energy-draining foods, particularly those that are acid-forming, such as dairy products, chocolate, wine, caffeine and sugar.

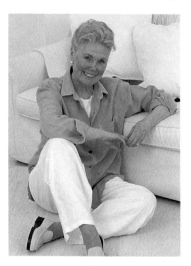

MAGNET THERAPY

Wearing a magnetic wristband is an increasingly popular self-help treatment for arthritis. It can improve the circulation and help to break down the toxic crystal deposits that have accumulated around the joints. The magnet should be worn on the inner wrist, next to the pulse point. Drinking plenty of water will help the body to flush out the toxins.

◀ ARTHRITIS CAN BE TREATED IN A NUMBER OF DIFFERENT WAYS TO ENSURE THAT YOUR LATER YEARS ARE ACTIVE AND LESS PAINFUL.

pain relief

Pain is the body's way of telling you that something is wrong and needs attention. It is often caused by an excess of energy of some sort. Energy treatments are based on rebalancing the energy rather than "killing" the pain.

Use crystals and colour healing to help reduce pain to manageable levels by releasing blocks in the subtle bodies and stimulating the body's healing mechanisms. In general, all cool colours – blue, indigo and violet – will help to calm painful areas and restore the natural flow of energy in a damaged area. Pink will calm aggravation and reduce fear. Placing pink stones at the 2nd and 3rd chakras will help to calm the mind and relax the body. Copper is well known for its ability to reduce inflammation and swellings, and some gemstones

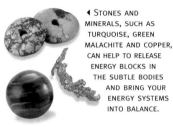

◀ STONES AND MINERALS, SUCH AS TURQUOISE, GREEN MALACHITE AND COPPER, CAN HELP TO RELEASE ENERGY BLOCKS IN THE SUBTLE BODIES AND BRING YOUR ENERGY SYSTEMS INTO BALANCE.

used for controlling pain have high concentrations of copper. Malachite, for instance, calms painful areas and is also a good absorber of negativity. Copper can be worn as a bracelet to help energy flow in the body.

▼ COLOUR VIBRATIONS CAN HELP TO SOOTHE PAIN. TURQUOISE HAS AN UPLIFTING HEALING ENERGY AND CAN CALM TROUBLED EMOTIONS.

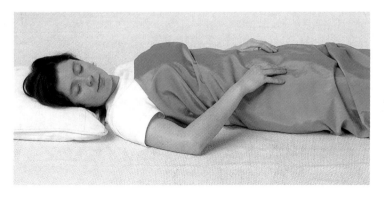

allergies and intolerances

True allergies are very rare, but over-sensitivity to certain foods or environmental factors is relatively common. These over-sensitivities or intolerances seem to be implicated in many common chronic health problems.

If you suspect that you may be suffering from an intolerance, the first step is to identify the key triggers that have a destabilizing effect on your immune system. Kinesiology, Vega testing and radionics will help you locate these. Use dowsing to check your response to common allergens. These include alcohol, caffeine, corn, dairy produce, soya, sugar, wheat, chocolate, tomatoes, moulds, pollen, house dust, animal hair, exhaust fumes, glues, paints, electro-magnetic radiation, fungicides and pesticides.

DESENSITIZATION STRATEGIES

The obvious strategy is to avoid contact with an allergen. This can mean making dietary changes and changing your washing detergent, for instance. Some allergens are unavoidable, however, in which case you need to reprogramme your immune system. Taking homeopathic dilutions of the offending substance, such as house dust or pollen, can help you to build up immunity. These remedies work rather like vaccinations, but on an energy level rather than a physical level.

▼ A USEFUL HOMEOPATHIC REMEDY FOR HAYFEVER IS EUPHRASIA (EYEBRIGHT), INDICATED WHEN EYES ARE RED AND SORE.

▼ IF YOU FIND YOU ARE INTOLERANT TO WHEAT PRODUCTS, IT WILL MEAN ELIMINATING CERTAIN TYPES OF BREAD FROM YOUR DIET.

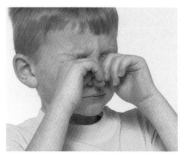

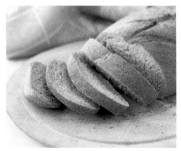

digestive problems

A healthy digestive system is crucial for health and wellbeing. Any digestive disorder, no matter how trivial it may seem, is a sign of an energy imbalance that needs to be taken seriously and treated accordingly.

Many digestive problems are linked to poor eating habits, food intolerance and emotional stress. If you suffer from frequent digestive problems, test for food allergens and eliminate any triggers from your diet. Many people are intolerant of wheat, corn and dairy products without realizing it. Eat a diet that is rich in energy-building foods, and avoid irritants such as tea, coffee, strong spices and alcohol. If your digestion is weak, raw food and elaborate meals with rich sauces are best avoided; instead, follow a plain diet that includes lightly steamed vegetables, chicken, fish, tofu and wholegrain rice. Drink plenty of water.

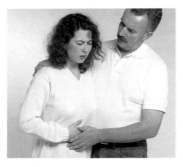

▲ MANY DIGESTIVE PROBLEMS ARE LINKED TO EMOTIONAL UPSETS.

BACH FLOWERS

When the problem is stress-related, taking Bach flower remedies can help to balance the mental and emotional bodies.

- Walnut: helps with a change in circumstances, such as a new job, moving house or divorce
- Scleranthus: constant dilemmas, unable to make decisions
- Vervain: wired up, unable to relax, chasing perfection
- Impatiens: impatient and also irritable, always in a hurry
- Crab apple: when revolted by food as well as eating; cleansing and detoxifying

> ### TIP
> A quick treatment for nausea and vomiting is to apply finger pressure to the acupuncture point that is situated about 3 cm (1¹/₄ in) above the wrist on the inside arm.

skin problems

The state of our health and wellbeing shows in the skin. Skin disorders can indicate problems with digestion or circulation or inadequate removal of toxins from the body. They may also be a visible sign of stress.

If your skin problem is stress-related, you need to find ways to release tension. Aerobic exercise will boost your energy and encourage the body to unwind. It also helps the body to release toxins. Drinking plenty of water helps to flush the toxins out of your system; starting the day with a glass of warm water will also encourage a sluggish digestive system to work more efficiently.

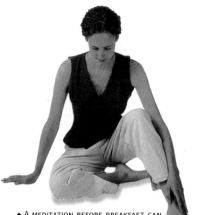

▲ A MEDITATION BEFORE BREAKFAST CAN BE VERY CALMING AND SOOTHING.

▼ IF YOU HAVE PROBLEM SKIN, TRY STARTING THE DAY WITH A GLASS OF WARM WATER RATHER THAN A CUP OF TEA OR COFFEE.

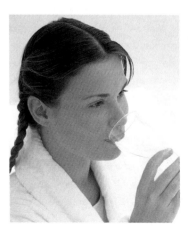

The redness, dryness and itching of many skin problems indicates excess heat. A cold shower will help to redress the balance, bringing the energy back inside the body and closing the pores.

COLOUR MEDITATION
A short meditation will set you up for the day; tune in and visualize which colours you need. Green, pale pink or blue are often helpful for aggravated skin conditions such as eczema or dermatitis.

PMS and menstrual cramps

Many women experience problems with menstruation. Fluctuating hormone levels, emotional stress and physical tension can unbalance the system, producing symptoms from extreme mood swings to severe physical pain.

Magnets can help to ease period pain by improving the flow of blood to the area. Apply the magnet midway between the pubic bone and the navel and leave in position for up to ten minutes. This should help to relieve the cramp. Alternatively use a Reiki hand treatment. Place one hand on the lower stomach and the other on the lower back; visualize healing Reiki energy flowing through your hand, dissolving any tension and bringing peace and wellbeing.

MOONTIME

The menstrual cycle mirrors the 28-day cycle of the moon. Your "moontime" is a time when your energy levels are low, and ideally you should spend more time relaxing so as to build your energy in preparation for the coming period. If you want to tune in to the cycles of the moon, moonstone is the ideal stone to work with. Moonstone helps to balance and relax emotional states. It can also have beneficial effects on all the body's fluid systems and ease tension in the abdominal area.

Apply moonstones to your body in a pattern that amplifies their potential for relaxing and healing. Place one stone at the top of your head, one on the front of each shoulder and one on each hip. Close your eyes and relax.

▼ TO TREAT PERIOD PAINS, CHANNEL HEALING ENERGY THROUGH YOUR HANDS WITH A RELAXING REIKI TREATMENT.

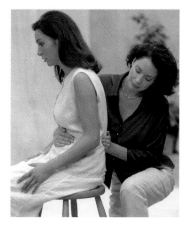

index

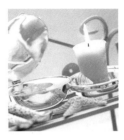

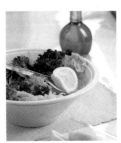